# How To Make The Best Smoothies At Home

by Martha Abdulhafiz

E-mail: smoothiedelite@gmail.com
Facebook page: How To Make The Best Smoothies At Home

# CONTENTS

# DEDICATION

To my beautiful family without you this will not be possible thanks for your patience.

My husband Jamee thank you for your support throughout these years. My lovely and brilliant children Nabila, Nadia and Omar. Love you guys So Much.

To my parents Jacques and Marie-Claire the world's best, supportive and loving parents.

# INTRODUCTION

## Let's Get Started

Whenever I'm in a quick pinch and need something nutritional that also tastes great, I break out my blender or juicer and grab some fruit and vegetables. I typically whip up a smoothie or juice when I'm in need of a pick-me-up or just a creamy, refreshing drink.

Now you might ask, "What is a smoothie"? A smoothie is a blended, sometimes sweetened, drink made from fruits and vegetables containing special add-ins such as flaxseeds, almond butter and honey just to name a few.

The great smoothie and juice phenomenon has taken the health world by storm. With new studies being released, more and more people are getting into the blended-food craze. In the weight loss world, smoothies can provide a variety of benefits to the human body and can help strengthen the immune system. Juices contribute to weight loss and can provide a lot of nutrients that most people don't get from their daily diets.

Before I was introduced to smoothies and juices, I used to resort to grabbing a processed, preservative-filled snack that didn't really fill me up or provided nutritional benefits. I only ate these kinds of foods because they were quick to grab and easy to buy in bulk at the store. But then, just like everyone else, I got caught up in the smoothie and juice phenomenon.

Both provide great benefits without all the added preservatives. I was shocked when I took the first sip of a smoothie and found it sweet, cool, and tasty. No sugar is needed to sweeten either of the drinks, as the natural sugars of the fruits and vegetables provide the necessary sweetness.

Smoothies and juices are both concoctions of fruits and vegetables. People often make smoothies and juices to get more nutrients into their daily diets or as refreshing drinks to cool down on a hot day. The only differences between the two are how you prepare them and what benefits you get from them.

Blending is a quick way to get a creamy drink that's also nutritious and full of vibrant taste. All you need is a handful of fruits or vegetables and a good, high quality blender. Blending takes the entire body of the fruit or vegetable and blends it into a creamy drink. While smoothies are more filling, they also contain the hard-to-digest fibers from the skin of the fruit or vegetable. These fibers are tough on our digestive systems, but it helps a slow release of nutrients into the bloodstream and helps avoid blood sugar spikes.

Juicing, on the other hand, is the squeezing of juice from a fruit or vegetable. It only squeezes out the valuable juices to form a refreshing, cool drink. It doesn't include the skin of the fruits or vegetable, making it easier on the digestive system because there's nothing to digest. However, juices aren't very filling and hunger pangs start shortly after.

However, both methods have a few drawbacks. Juicing and blending do not substitute complete meals and they are both dangerous to live solely off. Juicing is not a complete meal. Also, being on a smoothie regime for too long can endanger one's health. It is unwise to use juicing as a meal replacement unless you are under a special detox plan supervised by a medical doctor.

Also, it is advised that if you suffer from diabetes, you should consult your doctor. Starting a juicing detox plan while suffering with diabetes can be detrimental to health. Please consult a doctor if questions arise about juicing or blending.

For those interested in blending, the steps are simple. For blending, a good blender is required to puree the fruits and vegetables. It does not have to be an expensive piece of equipment, it just has to do the job.

To use a blender, add in vegetables or fruits and blend them together until the mixture is smooth and creamy. Juicing requires different equipment. Different from a blender, a juicer separates the juice from the pulp.

After getting caught up in this phenomenon, my go-to drink is a smoothie or juice. Usually, I whip up a quick, nutrient-packed smoothie before or after a rigorous workout to help repair my muscles. Smoothies and juices are great to sip on while lounging around the house or with a meal.

Smoothies and juices are also easily customizable to fit your needs, as they don't need specific ingredients. Take what you have in the fridge, throw it in a blender or a juicer, and you'll have a great treat. They're perfect for picky kids who are specific about what they like, and you'll be able to have a crisp drink that tastes good and provides great benefits.

Blending and juicing are both great ways to obtain more nutrients in a daily diet. No matter how you drink a smoothie or juice, you're getting the right ingredients in a cool and creamy concoction that can be customized to suit all tastes.

# CHAPTER ONE

## Juicing vs. Blending

Interested in getting all the nutrients your body needs while getting all the flavor your taste buds desire? Tired of eating all the processed foods and drinks that are filled with empty calories and artificial chemicals? Take a look at the popular trend that is sweeping the nation: juicing and blending.

Juicing and blending are both incredibly popular ways to get nutrients from your favorite fruits and vegetables, like strawberries, blueberries, and tomatoes. Both of them provide great health benefits, but people often bicker over which one is better for the body and digestive system. Both provide different advantages that can help build a better body and create a stronger immune system.

There are numerous ways to go about juicing, from crushing fruits and vegetables by hand to wide-scale extraction with mechanical equipment. Squeezing is, for the most part, a quick and easy way to get all the tasty and refreshing juice from strawberries, bananas, apples, and more, and it is completed through a machine called a juicer that presses out all the juice. Juicers remove the fibers from the skins of the fruits and vegetables, leaving a crisp, refreshing beverage.

Squeezing is not quite the same as purchasing squeeze in the store because it is concentrated without adding any preservatives or extra ingredients. Store-bought juice is loaded with extra preservatives and ingredients that a lot of people don't want. Juicing is frequently polished for dietary reasons or as a type of option for pharmaceuticals.

Becoming popular in the early 1990's, hobbies in juicing have taken off in the most recent decade because of various books, videos, and advertisements, and also, the fast spread because of the Internet.

Juicing gets rid of all the tough-to-digest fibers and only squeezes out what we want to drink. Imagine wanting to down a crisp glass of strawberry juice, only to find bits and pieces of the skin floating around. Yuck! With juicing, our systems don't have to work as hard to digest after we remove all the tough fibers. Juicing only gives us the juice that goes down easy on our digestive systems.

This method is preferred if you have a sensitive digestive system or want to get a lot of your daily nutrients in one glass. However, juicing often lacks the sustenance that blending has, resulting in hunger pangs shortly after consumption.

On the bright side, you can pack more servings of fruits and vegetables into a single serving of juice than you can into a smoothie. With smoothies, the process involves blending the entire strawberry, or the entire banana, or the entire body of food you're working with. This added fiber from the skin adds to the volume content. Because you don't have that fiber in juicing, you can add more servings in one glass than you can with blending.

Speaking of blending, this is a form of extraction that blends together the skin and the insides of your food of choice. While juicing merely extracts the juice, blending mixes up every part of the food. This is the most common way people make smoothies and more often than not, nothing needs to be added because the natural sugars of the ingredients make the concoction taste perfectly sweet. Yum!

But blending also keeps in all the fibers our digestive systems have trouble processing. This method is not recommended for people with sensitive digestive systems. But, while it slows down our systems, it is often more filling than juicing and can serve as a meal by itself.

Being hungry in the morning is the worst, but smoothies can help fill you up and keep you satisfied until lunch because of that added fiber. They help create an even release of nutrients into the bloodstream that avoids blood sugar spikes.

While juicing and blending provide different advantages, both are great ways to add extra nutrients to a daily diet. They can serve as a refreshing drink on a hot day, a quick on-the-go snack, or an energy-packed post-workout beverage.

Now, are you ready to get started?

# CHAPTER TWO

## What You Need

So now you've heard about the juicing and blending craze that has captured the hearts of millions across the nation. You're dying to try it, but don't know where to start or what you need. Read on to find out what kind of equipment you need to create the perfect smoothie or juice.

To get the most benefits from your juices and smoothies and save money, it's important to have the right equipment. This will help you get the most from your fresh strawberries, crisp mangos, and luscious tomatoes. Along with having the right equipment, it's important to have great quality, as poor quality equipment will run down easily. Having a good quality machine will prevent you from circulating through a round of machines when each one breaks.

For juicing, invest in a good quality juicer. This will help you get the most juice out of your succulent raspberries, juicy blackberries, and sweet blueberries. Nothing is worse than throwing all your fruits and vegetables into a juicer and having it give only a little bit of juice.

Personally, I suggest getting a premium cold-press juicer. A juicer like this will produce a great quality of juice and allow you to get more out of your tasty kiwis, tangy oranges, and mouthwatering pineapple. This saves you from having to buy more fruit and vegetables to fill up your glass each time you want to make a drink.

Investing in a great quality juicer will pay off. The machine will last longer and provide you with hundreds of glasses of juice. Make sure to buy a cold-press juicer instead of a centrifugal juicer, as cold-press juicers compress the fruits and vegetables to squeeze out their juice. You will get the most juice out this way.

The same goes for a blender. You want a good quality blender that will last for a long time. When buying a blender, you want one that is gentle on your produce and does not heat up the enzymes as it pulls apart the fibers. A good blender will evenly blend your fruits and vegetables while still maintaining the perfect taste you want to achieve.

Now that you're totally hooked on the juicing and blending craze and know what you need to get, go out there and make a great quality smoothie or juice!

# CHAPTER THREE

## Let's Make Smoothies (31 smoothies, one for every day)

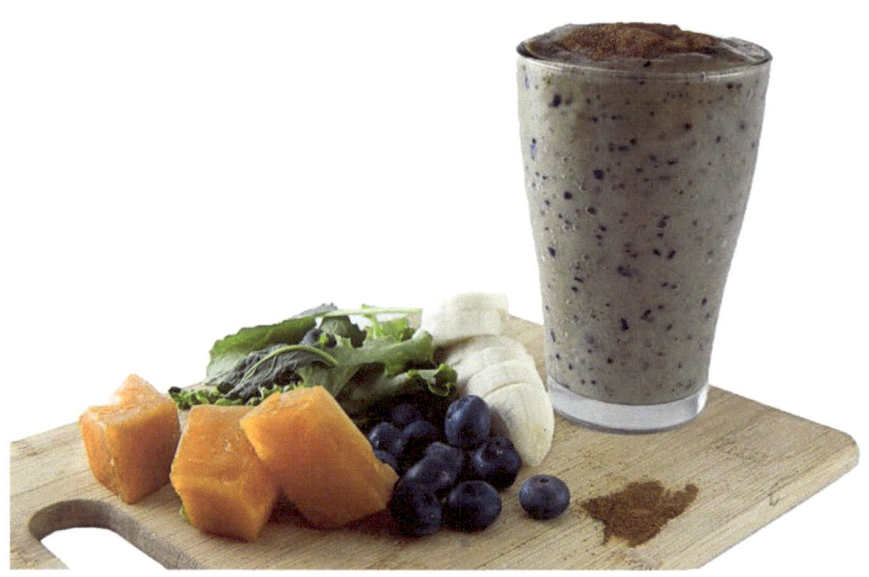

### *Day 1:Papaya-Banana Smoothie Delite*

½ cup papaya

¼ cup blueberries

1 small frozen banana (cut banana into one-inch chunks before freezing)

1 handful of kale

1 tbsp teaspoon coconut oil

1 inch thick fresh ginger crushed

1 tbsp flaxseeds

1 tbsp chia seeds

1 cup of almond milk or a milk of your choosing

4-5 ice cubes

Stevia (optional) only add stevia to your smoothies if you need to make your smoothie sweeter .

*Directions:*
1. Place all ingredients in blender. Always start with liquids first. Blend until smooth.
2. Pour in a fancy glass and serve immediately.
3. Sprinkle top with cinnamon or cardamom

Feel free to add more or less take something away or add something in. Invite your friends and family to have a smoothie date with you.

*** Have Fun with it ***

# *Day 2:Strawberry-Mango Layered Smoothie Delite*

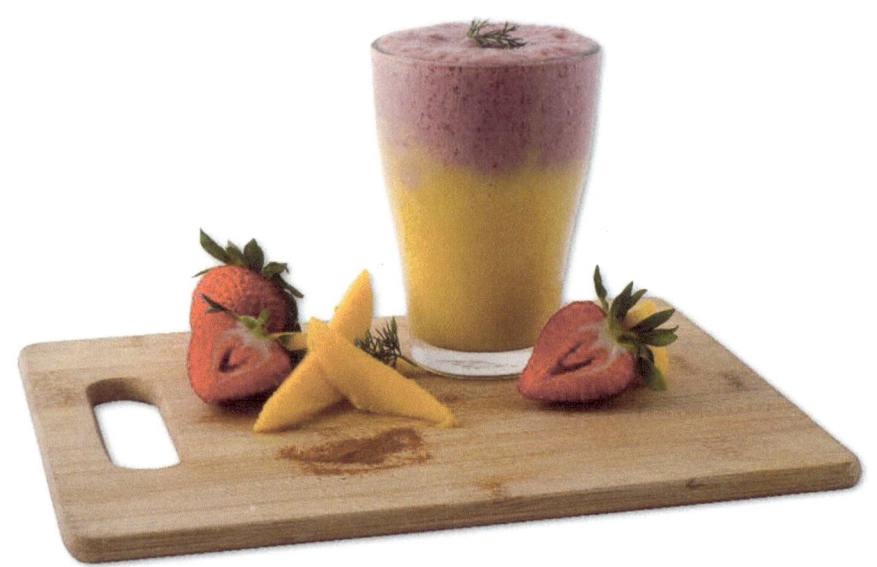

½ cup coconut milk

1 banana frozen (plan ahead)

1 mango fresh or frozen

10 strawberries

ice

*Mango Layer:*

1 Mango, peeled and cubed

½  cup of coconut milk

¼ cup crushed ice

*Strawberry Layer:*

10 strawberries cut and sliced

¼  cup crushed ice

*Directions:*

1. Blend mango in blender until smooth, add banana and crushed ice, and continue processing until fully blended. Pour into tall glass.

2. Rinse blender well. Blend strawberries until smooth. Add crushed ice and continue processing until fully blended. Pour on top of the mango layer and garnish with thyme.

# Day 3:Green Tea Smoothie Delite

½ cup of low fat Greek yogurt

1 cup of fresh mango or frozen

1 bag of green tea

1 half inch ginger crushed

4-5 ice cubes

*Directions:*

1. Brew tea in a bag for about 5 minutes. Then remove bag and let it sit at room temp until cool.
2. After cool add tea and ingredients in blender along with the other ingredients and blend until smooth.
3. Pour and serve. Garnish with mint leaves (optional)

# Day 4:Strawberry-Banana Protein Smoothie Delite

1 banana frozen

6 strawberries

1 scoop pea protein or any protein or oats

1 cup almond milk

4-5 ice cubes

*Directions:*

    1. Place all ingredients liquids first in to the blender. Blend all ingredients until smooth.

    2. Serve in a glass and sprinkle with chia seeds.

## *Day 5:Banana-Almond Smoothie Delite*

1 small frozen banana

1 cup almond milk

¾ cup almond

1 tbsp hemp seeds

4-5 ice cubes

1 inch thick ginger or you can use ground ginger

1 handful of kale or spinach (remove stems)

*Directions:*

1. Place all of the ingredients into the blender. Blend all ingredients until smooth.
2. Pour in a glass and sprinkle with cinnamon or a topping of your choosing.

## *Day 6:Pineapple-Coconut Smoothie Delite*

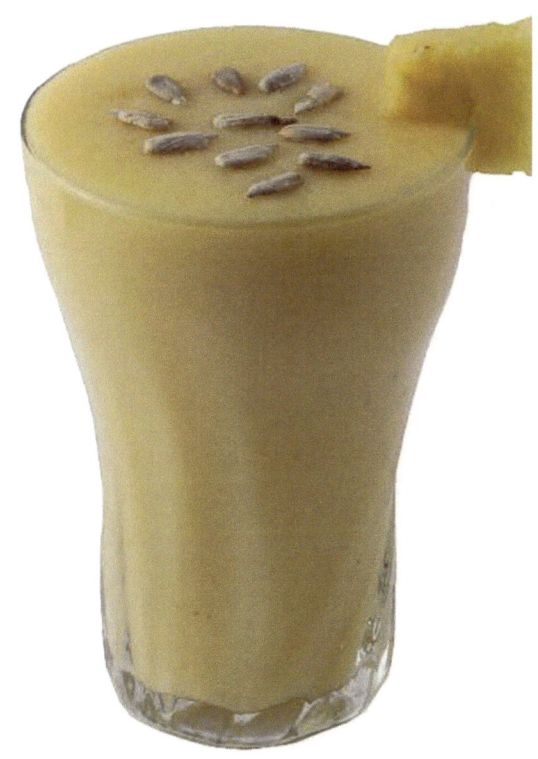

1 mango frozen or fresh

½ cup pineapple chunks

1 cup coconut milk or coconut water

Stevia (optional)

4-5 ice cubes

*Directions:*

1. Place all ingredients in. Blend all ingredients until smooth.
2. Pour in a glass and serve at once. Sprinkle with sunflower seeds.

# *Day 7:Granola Banana Smoothie Delite*

1 cup almond or soy milk

½ cup low-fat granola

1 frozen banana or ½ cup of dates

1 tbsp coconut oil

*Directions:*

      1. Place all ingredients. Blend all ingredients until smooth.

      2. Pour in a glass and sprinkle with wheat germs.

## *Day 8:Strawberry-Orange Smoothie Delite*

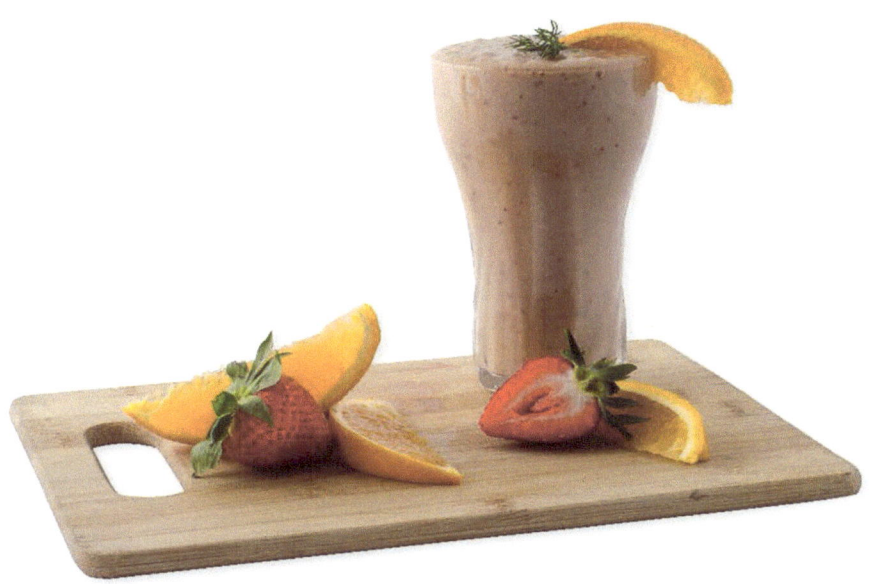

½ almond milk or yogurt

1 cup of fresh strawberries

2 -3 oranges (peeled and seeded)

1 scoop vanilla protein or oats

1 tbsp chia seeds

Stevia (optional)

4-5 ice cubes

*Directions:*

1. Place all ingredients in blender. Blend until smooth.
2. Pour in glass garnish with thyme and a slice of orange.  Serve immediately.

# *Day 9:Avocado-Green Smoothie Delite*

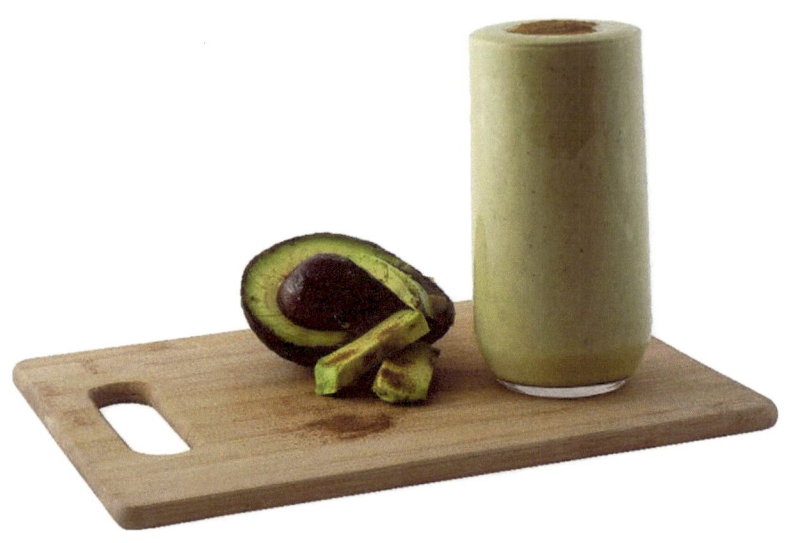

1 banana

1 cup coconut milk or almond milk

½ avocado

1 handful spinach or kale

1tbsp flax seeds

4-5 ice cubes

*Directions:*

     1. Place all ingredients in blender. Blend all ingredients until smooth.

     2. Pour in glass, sprinkle with cinnamon and serve right away.

# *Day 10:Very Berry Smoothie Delite*

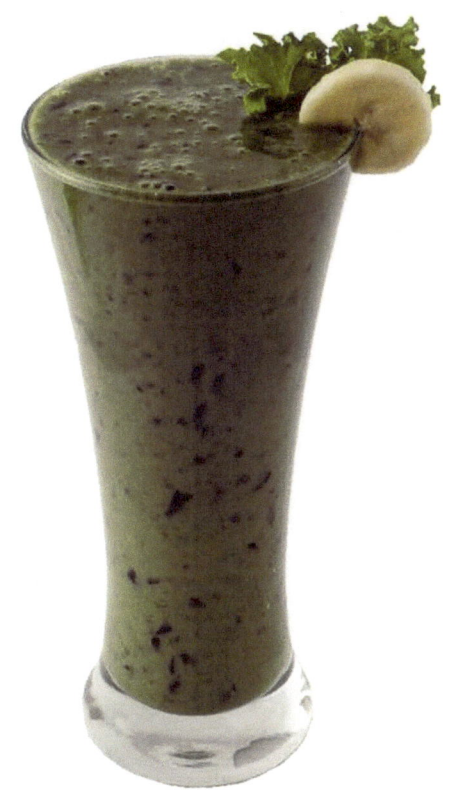

1 cup almond milk

½ banana

2 handfuls of kale

1 cup of frozen blueberries (freeze berries the night before)

1 cup of frozen blackberries

½ inch crushed ginger

½ teaspoon chia seeds

4-5 ice cubes (optional)

*Directions:*

1. Place all ingredients in blender. Blend until smooth.
2. Pour in a glass and garnish kale and a slice of banana.

# *Day 11:Peach-Guava Smoothie Delite*

½ cup of low fat Greek yogurt

½ cup of guava

½ banana or dates (both make great sweeteners)

1 tsp fresh lime

1 ½ tsp vanilla extract

2 peaches

1 tbsp coconut oil

4-5 ice cubes

*Directions:*

1. Place all ingredients in blender. Blend until smooth.
2. Pour in a glass and garnish with a piece of peach and enjoy!

# *Day 12:Peanut Butter-Banana Smoothie Delite*

1 cup of almond milk or soy milk

1 small frozen banana

1 tbsp wheat germ

2 tbsp peanut butter

¼ tsp vanilla

2-3 ice cubes (depending how cold you like your smoothies)

*Directions:*

1. Place all ingredients in blender. Blend until smooth.
2. Pour in a glass and top with cocoa snips. (Optional)

# Day 13:Raspberry-Honey Smoothie Delite

½ cup low fat Greek yogurt

1 tsp honey

¼ cup almond milk

1 tbsp coconut oil

1 tbsp flax seeds

4-5 ice cubes

*Directions:*
1. Place all ingredients in blender. Blend until smooth.
2. Pour in a glass, garnish with a few raspberries and serve.

# Day 14:Quinoa Smoothie Delite

½ cup quinoa cooked

1 frozen banana (cut up and frozen the night before)

1 cup of vanilla almond milk

½ inch

1 tbsp coconut oil

1 tbsp flax seeds

3-4 ice cubes (optional)

*Directions:*
1. Place all ingredients in blender. Blend until smooth.
2. Pour in a glass and sprinkle with cinnamon.

# *Day 15:Chocolate-Spinach Smoothie Delite*

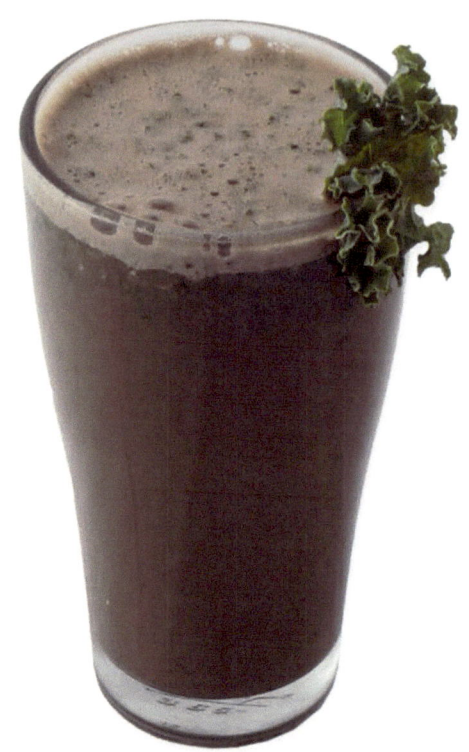

1 cup of almond milk

1 scoop of cacao

½ cup of rolled oats

1 handful of spinach or kale

½ tbsp chia seeds

½ an avocado

3-4 ice cubes

*Directions*:

1. Place all ingredients in blender. Blend until smooth.
2. Pour in a glass, garnish with a piece of kale and drink immediately.

# *Day 16:Coffee-Banana Smoothie Delite*

1 scoop protein

½ cup of almond milk/soy milk or a milk of your choosing

½ cup of coffee

1 frozen banana

1/3 cup of oats

1 tbsp coconut oil

3-4 ice cubes

*Directions:*
1. Place all ingredients in a blender. Blend until smooth.
2. Pour in a glass, serve and enjoy!

# *Day 17:Holiday Spice Galore Smoothie Delite*

1 cup almond milk

½ cup pumpkin

1 cup oats

½ tbsp of ginger, cloves, nutmeg and pumpkin spice

1/8 tsp vanilla extract

3-4 ice cubes

*Directions:*
1. Place all ingredients in a blender. Blend until smooth.
2. Serve in a fancy glass and remember to share your calories!

# *Day 18:Sweet Potato Pie Smoothie Delite*

1 cup of vanilla almond milk

½ cup of cooked and diced sweet potatoes

1 tbsp flax seed

1 tbsp chia seeds

3-4 ice cubes

*Directions:*

1. Place all ingredients in a blender. Blend until smooth
2. Pour in a glass, serve and top with cinnamon or cardamom

# *Day 19:Mango-Avocado Layered Smoothie Delite*

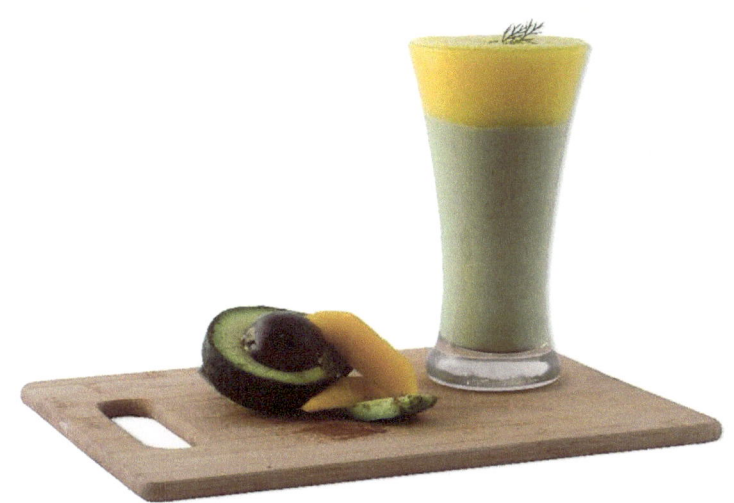

½ cup of almond milk

½ cup of Greek yogurt

½ a banana

1 avocado peeled and pitted

1 tbsp coconut oil

1 tbsp chia seeds grounded (optional)

1 tbsp flax seeds grounded (optional)

1 /8 tsp ginger grounded

Stevia (optional)

2-3 ice cubes

*Avocado & Banana Layer:*

1 avocado, peeled and pitted

½ a banana peeled and sliced

¼ cup of crushed ice

½ cup of almond milk

1 tbsp coconut oil

*Mango Layer:*

½ - 1 mango peeled and cubed

½ cup of Greek yogurt

1/8 tsp grounded ginger

¼ cup ice

*Directions:*

1. Blend avocado, almond milk, coconut oil until smooth. Add banana and crushed ice until smooth with no ice visible. Pour into a tall glass.
2. Rinse blender. Blend mango, Greek yogurt, and ginger until smooth. Add ice and process until blended well. Pour on top of the avocado layer. Garnish with dill weed or thyme.

# *Day 20:Watermelon Smoothie Delite*

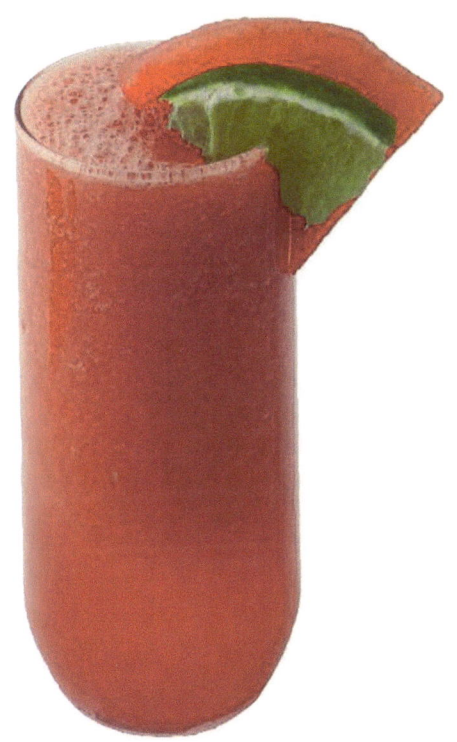

2 cups of watermelon cut up

1 ½ cups of coconut water

1 tbsp fresh lime

½ inch ginger grated

Stevia (optional)


*Directions:*

1. Place all ingredients and blend until smooth.
2. Pour in a tall glass and garnish with lime and a piece of watermelon.

# *Day 21:Coconut-Lime Smoothie Delite*

1 cup mangos (fresh or frozen)

1 banana

1 lime

1 cup coconut milk

1 tbsp coconut oil

1 tbsp flax seeds

1 tbsp chia seeds

*Directions:*
1. Place all ingredients in blender. Blend until smooth.
2. Take out 2 glasses and share with your spouse or friend. Cheers!

# *Day 22:Pear Smoothie Delite*

1 pear cut up

1 banana

1 cup almond milk or soy milk

1 tbsp chia seeds

1 inch thick crushed fresh ginger

1 tsp cinnamon

*Directions:*
1. Place all ingredients in blender. Blend until smooth.
2. Pour and serve. Top with cardamom.

# Day 23:Plum Smoothie Delite

½ cup of non-fat Greek yogurt

1 plum pitted and chopped

1 peach pitted, removed, then chopped

1 nectarine pit removed and chopped

½ cup of frozen blueberries

*Directions:*

1. Place all ingredients in blender. Blend until smooth.
2. Pour in a glass and enjoy!

# Day 24:Honey-Cantaloupe Smoothie Delite

½ cup of non-fat plain Greek yogurt

1 tbsp honey

1 tbsp flax seeds

½ cup of cantaloupe

4-5 ice cubes

*Directions:*

1. Place all ingredients in blender. Blend until smooth.
2. Pour and serve.

# Day 25:Pina Colada Smoothie Delite

½ cup of fresh or frozen pineapples

1 tsp honey

½ cup of almond milk

1 tsp coconut oil (optional)

½ tbsp chia seeds

½ tbsp flax seeds

3-4 ice cubes

\

*Directions*:

1. Place all ingredients. Blend until smooth.
2. Pour in a glass and sprinkle a topping of your choice.

# *Day 26:Cucumber Smoothie Delite*

1 cup of coconut water

½ cup of spinach

½ a cucumber

3 celery stalks

1 apple peeled, cored and cut up

1 inch piece of ginger crushed

3-4 ice cubes

*Directions:*

1. Place all ingredients in blender. Blend until smooth.
2. Pour in glass and enjoy immediately.

# *Day 27:Very Berry Smoothie Delite*

½ cup of cherries (pitted)

½ cup of non-fat Greek yogurt

2 tbsps of honey

1 tbsp flax seeds

3-4 ice cubes

*Directions:*
1. Place all ingredients in a blender. Blend until smooth.
2. Pour in a fancy glass and enjoy.

# Day 28:Beet Smoothie Delite

1 cup of coconut water

1 orange peeled and seeded

1 lime

1 small beet

3-4 ice cubes

*Directions:*
1. Place all ingredients in a blender. Blend until smooth.
2. Pour in a glass and drink immediately!

# Day 29:Island Soursop Smoothie Delite

1 ripe soursop

1 cup of almond vanilla milk

1 tsp grated nutmeg

1 tsp ginger grated

1 tbsp fresh lime juice

1 tsp vanilla extract

1 tbsp chia seeds

1 tbsp flax seeds

3-4 ice cubes

*Directions:*

1. Wash soursop. Pour water in large bowl, use hands to remove all seeds. Pour mixture into blender while adding all other ingredients.
2. Pour in a glass with a dash of nutmeg and ginger.

# Day 30:Pumpkin Spiced Smoothie Delite

1 cup of almond milk

1 cup of pumpkin

1 banana or a cup of dates

1 tbsp chia seeds

1 tbsp flax seeds

1 tbsp coconut oil

½ tsp cinnamon

1 inch thick ginger crushed

3-4 ice cubes

*Directions:*

1. Place all ingredients in a blender. Blend until smooth.
2. Pour in a glass, serve, sprinkle with cinnamon or cardamom and enjoy!

# *Day 31:Mango Lassi Smoothie Delite*

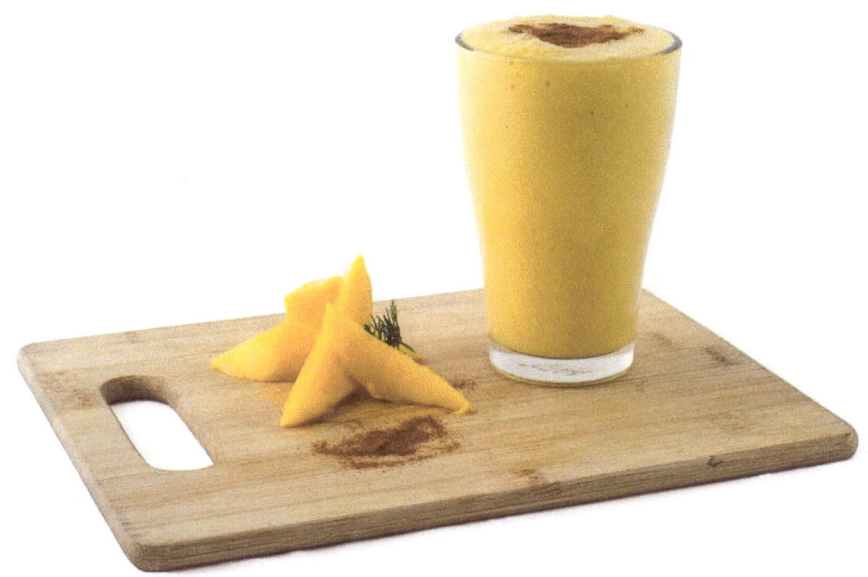

1 ½ cups of diced fresh mango

1 ½ cups of plain non-fat Greek yogurt

1 tbsp lime juice

½ inch ginger crushed

3-4 ice cubes

*Directions:*

1. Place all ingredients except ice in a blender. Blend until smooth. Then add ice and continue the blending process until completely smooth
2. Pour in a fancy glass. Sprinkle with cinnamon or cardamom. Share your calories with a loved one or friend. Enjoy!

# CHAPTER FOUR

## You Are What You Eat (superfoods)

Have you ever heard the saying you are what you eat? Health and wellness is closely associated to the types of foods we choose to put in our bodies.

Fruit and vegetables are good for us. Whether raw, squeezed or crushed, studies show that fruit can help keep our hearts healthy and reduces our risk of some types of cancer.

Health experts recommend that we should all have at least 5 portions of fruit and vegetables every day (around 400g), but only a third of adults actually achieve that number.

The experts at the Department of Health have officially confirmed that 100% fruit juices and smoothies count towards your 5-a-day; one 150ml glass of fruit juice can count as one of your 5 portions.

Smoothies are a great way of getting the 5-a-day recommended by health professionals without feeling like we are forcing ourselves to eat more fruit and vegetables throughout the day. Simply blend and drink. It's that simple.

However, smoothies and juices should not be a replacement every day for your intake of fruit and vegetables. You should also eat fruit and vegetables separately to ensure you get all the goodness without any of the breakdown from blending or juicing.

Milk or yogurt based smoothies have naturally more calories, but they also have a nice amount of protein. The advantage is that vitamin C that is present in fruits or vegetables is needed to absorb calcium from the milk or yogurt, so the amount of calcium absorbed is relatively high. Another advantage is that the combination of protein and sugar keeps you full for longer; approximately twice longer than a fruit smoothie which is water based.

Two very important nutritious intakes from smoothies are Vitamin C and Fiber:

**Vitamin C**

Vitamin C is classed as an antioxidant, along with vitamins A and E. Vitamin C is fundamentally important to prevent other elements from damaging our cells. Basically, Vitamin C protects our cells from oxidative stress (a bit technical there, but just know that it is important). Using fruit and vegetables enriched with Vitamin C for smoothies and juices is an excellent way of getting it in to our systems.

**Fiber**

This is an essential part of our diet, it helps to regulate our digestive system, and just like fruit and vegetables we just aren't getting enough. By including fruits and vegetables in smoothies, skin and all, we get all the goodness of the fruit or vegetable including the thick skin which in its purest form contains lots of fiber.

But it's important to note: nutritional value of juices and smoothies is kept when they are fresh, but as time goes on, more vitamins and antioxidants break down and it is no longer useful to the body. Also some juices don't contain the same amount of fiber as eating the whole fruit or vegetable.

*Here is a list of superfoods that are filled fiber, vitamins, minerals and other nutrients:*

- **Aloe Vera** has anti-inflammatory anti-bacterial and antifungal properties

- **Avocados** is classified as a fruit. They are filled with vitamins, beta carotene, potassium, magnesium, fiber and fat. The GOOD fat. Monosaturated fat. The one that will not raise your bad cholesterol level.

- **Bananas** can soothe your upset stomach, stop diarrhea and help suppress appetite and contains plenty of fiber and pectin. And a great source of potassium.

- **Bee pollen** increases stamina and energy level.

- **Blueberries** are filled with anti-oxidants that helps protect your brain. Blueberries are packed with vitamin C. Blueberries have vitamin A and beta carotene that helps prevent infections, heart disease and cancer.

- **Brewer's yeast** is a great source of vitamin B-12.

- **Cranberries** are filled with vitamin C and fiber. Helps with urinary tract infections.

- **Flax oil** boosts immune systems

- **Grapefruits.** Half of a grapefruit contains 70 percent vitamin C, contains cancer fighting flavonoids and potassium. Grapefruits do not interact well with some prescription drugs so talk to your doctor before you include then in your daily diet

- **Kiwifruit** has twice the amount of vitamin C of an orange. It also has lots of fiber, potassium and magnesium.

- **Mango,** an exotic fruit. Mostly found in tropical areas, one of my favorite fruits, Mangos are packed with beta carotene. One cup of mango has 160 percent of your daily vitamin A, 95 percent of C and 14 percent of B6.

- **Oranges** are filled with vitamin C. Oranges also have the fiber pectin that helps reduce bad cholesterol. They also contain potassium.

- **Raspberries** have lots of antioxidants 50 percent more cancer fighting agents than strawberries and 52 percent of your daily vitamin C.

- **Raw chocolate** slows aging process and is packed with antioxidants.

- **Strawberries** contain 140 percent of your daily vitamin C and lots of fiber.

- **Yogurt** or **Kefir** fights bacterial infections and helps digestion.

By adding these superfoods in your diet you can help fight disease, maintain your weight and live a longer healthy life.

It is also important you understand some of the important nutritional values of juices, below is a list of some of the recommended juices.

**Nutritional value of juices:**

- **Tomato juice** – contains a very large amount of vitamin C and lycopene, which helps prevent prostate cancer and cataracts.

- **Grapefruit juice** – contains antioxidants that reduce cholesterol and blood lipids.

- **Pomegranate juice** – contains polyphenols were found to be effective against many types of cancer.

- **Cranberry juice** – contains substances that prevent adherence to the bladder bacteria and helps prevent bladder infections.

- **Wheat grass juice** – contains chlorophyll which helps build haemoglobin, iron and protein. Because it is very bitter, it is better to mix it with orange juice or carrot juice (in a ratio of 1 to 1).

- **Carrot juice** – rich in beta-carotene, anti-cancer and strengthen the immune system.

- **Apple juice** – is effective against asthma.

- **Celery juice** – contains calcium and is effective against osteoporosis.

- **Parsley juice** – contains iron, folic acid, helps prevent oedema and renal function (since it has a diuretic effect).

- **Prune juice** – helps the proper functioning of the digestive system and helps against constipation.

# CHAPTER FIVE

## Tips For Making The Best Smoothies

There are a number of tips I have learned throughout the years I have been making smoothies. Below you will find my favorite ones.

- Plan ahead- shop at your local farmers markets or local farms for fresh fruits and vegetables. You can also use canned or frozen ones. Fresh is always best though.
- Wash and cut up your fruits and veggies ahead of time
- You can extend the life of your fruits (berries last longer) by filling the sink up with water and a ½ cup of vinegar for a 10 minute soak, pat dry and refrigerate. They will last for weeks!
- Freeze your fruits, which makes for a thicker consistency.
- Use tea as a base in your smoothie for a boost instead of milk, water or juice.
- Start off with liquids first.
- Use the lowest speed and then slowly work your way up to the higher speeds.
- If you have a thin smoothie add more frozen ingredients.
- If you have a smoothie that is too thick add more liquids.
- For a boost powered protein, use soy, whey or pea, however, these are considered processed foods. You should probably limit your consumption of these proteins.
- Use coconut water as a base for your smoothies. Coconut is filled with energy boosting goodness. And is also packed with electrolytes
- Oats add bulk to your smoothies and keep you filled up and is a rich source of important minerals.
- Power foods for a power boost include maca, cocoa, goji berries, hemp, and, coconut oil, nuts, seeds, spirulina and acai berries.

- Spices can really add a kick to your smoothies. Experiment with different ones. My favorites are cinnamon, cayenne pepper, ginger and nutmeg
- Healthy fats like avocado and hemp oil are great.
- Liquids to have on hand include almond milk sweetened and unsweetened, coconut water and yogurt.
- Use lime or lemon to help cut down on the bitterness of your bitter veggies.
- Use mostly fruits for sweetening your smoothies or juices, like dates, bananas and honey.
- Feel free to experiment and be adventurous with different fruits and vegetables. You can change a recipe to your own liking.
- Use what is in season.
- Be frugal with your fruits and sweet veggies that contain more sugars. Put more greens to balance the sugars.
- If you have to store your left over smoothie make sure you store it in a glass container and fill it up to the top of the glass in an airtight container this prevents the air from oxidizing. It can make your smoothies less nutritious. It is best to freeze your extra smoothie or left overs in an ice tray. You can throw in a cup when you are headed to the gym. By the time I am finished with my workout it is melted down into a juicy and frosty smoothie.
- Add lemon juice to your smoothie as this extra vitamin c will help prevent oxidization.
- Have fun with your friends and family. Kids love to be involved in making smoothies. What a lovely way to introduce them to healthy eating and drinking. And let me know how you did!!! You can do this via my facebook page How To Make The Best Smoothies At Home or contacting me at smoothiedelite@gmail.com.

# CHAPTER SIX

## Icing On The Cake (toppings and add-ins)

Making a great nutritious smoothie is dependent on a lot of things including what you use as a topping or add-ins. You can simply alter any recipe to your taste and liking and perhaps to a health benefit you wish to take advantage of. Simply add one or more of these to your smoothie for a super health or flavor kick.

-**Fresh fruits** and **vegetables.**
-**Nuts** a good source of protein.
-**Hemp seeds** a vegan protein with a nutty flavor.
-**Flaxseed** high fiber, protein packed with omega-3s.
-**Wheat germs** a dietary fiber.
-**Chia seeds** protein rich and contains lots of fiber and controls blood sugar.
-**Sunflower seeds** for a boost of copper, magnesium and selenium.
-**Ginger** helps in absorption and is used as a spice.
-**Coconut oil** increases your energy and is loaded with saturated fats.
-**Cinnamon** regulates blood sugar and is a natural food preservative.
-**Turmeric** is a powerful anti-inflammatory.
-**Spinach** is a superfood loaded with nutrients, but is low in calories. It lowers the risk of cancer and lowers blood pressure.
-**Kale** is high in fiber, low in calories. One cup is only 5 calories.
-**Papaya** contains unique protein digesting enzymes including papain and chymopapain.
-**Mint** promotes digestion, mint is effective in relieving nausea. Mint is also effective in clearing up congestion of the nose, throat and lungs.

-**Almond butter** rich in antioxidants, good for the heart, controls blood sugar and lowers blood pressure.

-**Peanut butter** is packed with monounsaturated fats, powerful antioxidant, vitamin E, potassium and magnesium.

-**Stevia** is a sweetener and sugar substitute made from the leaves of the plant Stevia rebaudiana.

-**Honey** prevents cancer and heart disease, reduces cough and throat irritation, regulates blood sugar and is a probiotic.

-**Wheat grass,** fresh or powered, boosts energy levels

It is important that you know your body and that you are aware what your body likes and doesn't like. If you have a sensitive digestive system then becoming heavily reliant on smoothies as a way of getting your health needs isn't a good idea, as previously discussed the fiber in the skin of the fruits can be too much. But a balance between smoothies and juices could work for you. It is equally important that you know if you have any allergies or reactions to certain foods as well as knowing whether a combination of fruit and vegetables works well for your stomach and health.

You can become an expert on your health through the use of smoothies by simply reading and re-reading this book, gleaning all of the tips and taking all of the nutrition and health information regarding certain fruits and vegetables and becoming a pro smoothie maker.

Remember what you put in your smoothies can either break you or make you. I mean this literally.

# CONCLUSION

Well, now you already know a lot around the health craze that's sweeping the world. This would be the blending and juicing trend, and it's gotten everyone hooked, including you!

After reading this book, you now know the actual difference between juicing and blending and are also eager to try it on your own. If you didn't catch everything before, I'll recap everything for you.

Juicing is the extraction of juice via delicious fruit and veggies, like tangy melons, sweet strawberries, and juicy tomatoes. With juicing, you'll be able to extract only the tasty juice without drinking in all the skin. This procedure is highly suggested for those who have irritable and sensitive digestive systems, as it removes the fiber from the skin and gives you just the smooth juice.

Juicing is a great way to get all the nutrients your body craves in one single glass. Juices are customizable, so you can juice just about any fruit or vegetable to create a great-tasting drink, catered in your own tastes.

But even though juices usually are tasty, savory, and refreshing on a hot evening, they aren't suitable meal replacements. Unless the juice is made by a medical professional, juices should not be consumed as a complete meal.

Blending, alternatively, blends the entire fruit or vegetable, skin and all, to make a frothy, creamy drink. Smoothies usually are recommended as breakfast drinks, since they contain a lot of fiber that will keep you full for hours. Since blending involves blending the skin of the fruit or vegetable, the fiber count rises, resulting in a thicker blend that will keep you satisfied.

Also with blending, you can pop in a handful of blueberries, among other healthy fruits, and you've got a great morning shake. If you favor veggies instead, throw in a few tomatoes and some other healthy vegetables, and you've got a flavorful, savory vegetable smoothie that will keep you full for long periods of time.

Just like juices, smoothies aren't safe for you to drink as a complete meal, unless you've been given clearance by a medical specialist. Smoothies and juices carry plenty of nutrients and give the body great benefits, but can only be meal replacements if made by a medical specialist.

Making smoothies in addition to juices are actually pretty quick. All you will need is the appropriate equipment so you can make a smoothie or maybe juice quickly. All you will need is a good blender or maybe juicer in addition too and you're ready to go!

Smoothies and juices are ideal for drinks on-the-go in the mornings, or as a pick-me-up from a rigorous workout. After workouts, you could create a protein-filled smoothie or juice that will refuel your muscles. They're also great beverages for afternoons when it's so sizzling outside and you need a refreshing, quick beverage to cool you down.

Believe it or not, smoothies and juices aren't just for you. You can make them for friends and family, as well as picky kids. For those kids with picky tastes, you can let them customize their own smoothie or juice! Just let them pick out their own fruits and vegetables and throw them in a blender or juicer, and you've got a cool treat that will satisfy their picky tastes.

Now, you're probably hooked into the smoothie and juice craze that's sweeping the nation, as well as the rest of the globe. If somehow you're not totally hooked, read the book again.

After reading this book, you've got all the information you need in order to create your own smoothie or juice. All it takes is your favorite succulent fruits or vegetables, a good quality blender or juicer, and a few minutes out of your day.

After practicing a few times, you'll soon become the master of the blender or juicer! Just pick up the ingredients from your local grocery store and get blending or juicing!

www.ingramcontent.com/pod-product-compliance
Lightning Source LLC
Chambersburg PA
CBHW040326010626
45792CB00024B/2159